DR. SEB

Natural ways to detox the liver, Reverse High Blood Pressure and cure Diabetes and Herpes to enjoy good health long life

Clarion Anderson

copyright@2020

Table of contents

CHAPTER ONE 3

   INTRODUCTION TO DR SEBI DIET 3

   What is the Dr. Sebi Diet? 4

CHAPTER TWO 7

   HOW DO I FOLLOW THE DR. SEBI DIET 7

CHAPTER THREE 11

   WOULD IT BE ABLE TO HELP LOSE WEIGHT? 11

CHAPTER FOUR 14

   LIKELY BENEFITS OF THE DR. SEBI DIET 14

CHAPTER FIVE 17

   DRAWBACKS OF THE DR. SEBI DIET 17

CHAPTER SIX 23

   FOODS TO CONSUME 23

CHAPTER SEVEN 26

   FOODS TO AVOID 26

CHAPTER EIGHT 28

   DR SEBI SAMPLE MENU 28

CHAPTER NINE 33

   DR SEBI FOOD LIST 33

   IN CONCLUSION 41

CHAPTER ONE

INTRODUCTION TO DR SEBI DIET

The Dr. Sebi diet, is also referred to as Dr. Sebi alkaline diet, is a plant-based eating routine created by the late Dr. Sebi.

It's professed to revive your cells by wiping out harmful material through alkalizing your blood.

The Dr. Sebi Diet depends on eating a short rundown of selected meals that is approved alongside other food supplements.

This book will be revealing the advantages and disadvantages of the Dr. Sebi diet and whether logical proof backs up its health and wellbeing claims.

What is the Dr. Sebi Diet?

This diet depends on the African Bio-Mineral Balance hypothesis and was created by a renowned and selt taught herbalist called Alfredo Darrington Bowman, He is generally known as Dr. Sebi. In spite of his name, Dr. Sebi was not a trained medical doctor neither does he hold a PhD.

He planned this eating routine for any individual who wishes to naturally treat ailments or inhibit diseases and improve their general wellbeing without depending on orthodox Western medication.

As per Dr. Sebi, diseases or ailments is an aftereffect of bodily fluid develop in a region of your body. For instance, a development of bodily fluid in the lungs is pneumonia, while surplus bodily fluid in the pancreas is diabetes.

He contends that ailments can't exist in environment that is alkaline and it starts to happen when your body turns out to be excessively acidic.

By carefully following his meal plan and utilizing his restrictive exorbitant supplements, he vows to reestablish your body's characteristic alkaline state and detoxify your unhealthy body.

Initially, Dr. Sebi guaranteed that this eating routine could fix conditions like AIDS, sickle cell sickliness, leukemia, and lupus. In any case, after a 1993 claim, he was requested to cease making such cases.

The eating routine comprises of a particular rundown of endorsed vegetables, natural products, grains, nuts, seeds, oils, and spices. Products from animals are not allowed, the Dr. Sebi diet is viewed as a vegetarian diet.

Sebi guaranteed that for your body to recuperate itself, you should follow the eating routine reliably for a very long time, for a life time if possible.

At long last, while numerous individuals demand that the program has recuperated them, no logical examinations uphold these cases.

In summary

The Dr. Sebi diet stresses that food intakes and enhancements or supplements that evidently decline illness causing bodily fluid by accomplishing an alkaline state in your body.

CHAPTER TWO

HOW DO I FOLLOW THE DR. SEBI DIET

The Dr. Sebi diet guidelines are listed below and they are to be adhered to strictly.

As indicated by Dr. Sebi's health and nutritional guide, you should observe these key principles:

- Rule 1. The only foods that you must consume are the ones listed on the nutritional guide

- Rule 2. Drink 1 gallon (3.8 liters) of water each day.

- Rule 3. Take Dr. Sebi's enhancements or supplements an hour prior to drugs.

- Rule 4. Animal products are not allowed.

- Rule 5. No liquor is permitted.

- Rule 6. Keep away from wheat items and just devour the "characteristic developing grains" recorded in the guide.

- Rule 7. Abstain from utilizing a microwave to avoid destroying your food nutrient.

- Rule 8. Stop taking canned or seedless fruits.

There are no particular supplement rules. In any case, this eating routine is low in protein, as it precludes beans, lentils, and creature and soy items. Protein is a significant supplement required for solid muscles, skin, and joints.

Also, you're required to buy Dr. Sebi's cell food items, which are supplements that guarantee to purge your body and sustain your cells.

It's prescribed to purchase the "comprehensive" package, which contains 20 unique items that are professed to purify and reestablish your whole body at the quickest rate possible.

Other than this, no particular recommendations are given

Besides this, rather, you're required to arrange any enhancement that coordinates your wellbeing concerns.

For instance, the "Bio Ferro" cases guarantee to treat liver issues, scrub your blood, support resistance, advance weight reduction, help stomach related problems, and increment generally prosperity.

Besides, the enhancements don't contain a total rundown of supplements or their amounts, making it hard to tell whether they will meet your everyday needs.

In Summary;

The Dr. Sebi diet has eight fundamental principles that must be followed. They for the most part center on avoiding animal products, super handled food, and taking his exclusive enhancements.

CHAPTER THREE

WOULD IT BE ABLE TO HELP LOSE WEIGHT?

While Dr. Sebi's eating regimen isn't intended for weight reduction, you may get more fit in the event that you follow it.

This diet plan doesn't encourage the consumption of western diet as it is known to contain high ultra-processed foods and loaded with salt, sugar, fat and calories.

Rather, it advances a natural, plant-based eating routine. Contrasted and the Western eating routine, the individuals who follow a plant-based eating routine will in general have lower paces of dealing with obesity and reduces chances of heart diseases.

A study that took a year taking 65 individuals as a case study found that the individuals who followed an unlimited complete food, low-fat, plant-based eating routine lost fundamentally more weight than individuals who didn't follow the eating routine.

At the half year point, those on the eating routine had lost a normal of 26.6 pounds (12.1 kg), contrasted and 3.5 pounds (1.6 kg) in the benchmark group.

Besides, most meals on this eating routine are low in calories, aside from nuts, seeds, avocados, and oils. Along these lines, regardless of whether you ate an enormous volume of affirmed nourishments, it's far-fetched that it would bring about an excess of calories and lead to weight gain.

In any case, extremely low-calorie slims down for the most part can't be kept up long haul. The vast majority who follow these eating plans recover the weight once they continue a typical eating design.

Since this eating routine doesn't indicate amounts and bits, it's hard to state whether it will give enough calories to maintainable weight reduction.

In summary

The Dr. Sebi diet isn't intended for weight reduction however is exceptionally low in calories and reduces the intake of processed foods. Along these lines, you may lose some weight in the event that you follow this eating plan.

CHAPTER FOUR

LIKELY BENEFITS OF THE DR. SEBI DIET

One advantage of the Dr. Sebi diet is that it emphasizes greatly on foods that are plant-based.

The eating routine advances eating countless vegetables and fruits, which are high in fiber, nutrients, minerals, and plant mixes.

The diets that are known to lower inflammation and oxidative stress and offer protection against diseases are diets with lots of vegetables and fruits. This also serves as insurance against several infections and diseases.

A research involving 65,226 individuals, the individuals who ate at least 7 servings of vegetables and fruits every day had a 25% and 31% lower rate of cancer and heart related diseases separately.

Moreover, a great many people are not eating enough produce. In a 2017 report, 9.3% and 12.2% of individuals met the proposals for vegetables and fruit, separately.

In addition, the Dr. Sebi diet advances eating fiber-rich entire grains and solid fats, for example, nuts, seeds, and plant oils. These nourishments have been connected to a lower danger of heart related illnesses.

At last, foods that drastically reduce super prepared nourishments are related with better diet quality in all.

In Summary

The Dr. Sebi diet stresses eating supplement rich vegetables, natural products, entire grains, and solid fats, which may diminish your danger of coronary illness, cancer, and inflammation.

CHAPTER FIVE

DRAWBACKS OF THE DR. SEBI DIET

Remember that there are a few downsides to this eating plan.

Strongly Restrictive

A significant drawback of Dr. Sebi's diet is that it constraints several food types, for example, all products from animals, wheat, beans, lentils, and numerous sorts of vegetables and fruits.

Indeed, it's exacting to such an extent that it just permits explicit kinds of fruits. For instance, you're permitted to eat cherry or plum tomatoes yet not different assortments like beefsteak or roma tomatoes.

In addition, following such a prohibitive eating plan isn't

agreeable and may prompt a negative relationship with food, particularly since this eating routine criticizes nourishments that are not recorded in the nutrition guide.

At last, this eating routine energizes other negative practices, for example, utilizing supplements to accomplish satisfaction. Given that supplements are not a significant wellspring of calories, this case further drives unhealthy and strange patterns of eating.

Needs Protein and Other Essential Nutrients

The nourishments recorded in Dr. Sebi's food guide can be a superb wellspring of nutrition.

In any case, none of the allowed foods are acceptable sources of protein, a fundamental supplement for skin structure, muscle development, and the creation of compounds and hormones.

Just walnuts, Brazil nuts, sesame seeds, and hemp seeds are allowed, which aren't extraordinary sources of protein. For instance, 1/4 cup (25 grams) of pecans and 3 tbsp (30 grams) of hemp seeds give 4 grams and 9 grams of protein, separately.

To meet your day by day protein needs, you would need to eat amazingly huge amounts of these nourishments.

Despite the fact that nourishments in this eating routine are high in specific supplements, for example, beta carotene, potassium, and nutrients C and E, they're low in omega-3, iron, calcium, and nutrients D and B12, which are normal supplements of worry for those after a carefully plant-based eating plan.

Dr. Sebi's expresses that specific fixings in his supplements are exclusive and not recorded. This is worrisome, as it's hazy which supplements you're getting and how a lot, making it hard to tell whether you'll meet your everyday supplement needs.

Not Based on Real Science

Perhaps the greatest worry with Dr. Sebi's eating plan approach is the absence of logical proof to help it.

He expresses that the nourishments and supplements in his eating plan control corrosive creation in your body.

Nonetheless, the human body carefully directs corrosive base parity to keep blood pH levels somewhere in the range of 7.36 and 7.44, normally making your body marginally alkaline.

In uncommon cases, for example, ketoacidosis from diabetes, blood pH can leave this reach. This can be lethal without quick clinical consideration.

At long last, research has demonstrated that your eating routine may somewhat and briefly change your urine pH however not blood pH. Thusly, following Dr. Sebi's eating routine won't make your body more alkaline.

In Summary

The Dr. Sebi diet may advance weight reduction however is prohibitive and low in numerous fundamental supplements, for example, protein, omega-3, iron, calcium, and nutrients D and B12. It likewise disregards your body's normal capacity to manage blood pH levels.

CHAPTER SIX

FOODS TO CONSUME

Dr. Sebi's food guide lists explicit nourishments permitted on the eating plan, including:

- Fruits: apples, melon, currants, dates, figs, elderberries, papayas, berries, peaches, delicate jam coconuts, pears, plums, cultivated key limes, mangoes, thorny pears, cultivated melons, Latin or West Indies soursop, tamarind.

- Vegetables: avocado, ringer peppers, desert flora bloom, chickpeas, cucumber, dandelion greens, kale, lettuce (aside from ice shelf), mushrooms (aside from shiitake), okra, olives, ocean vegetables, squash, tomatoes (just cherry and plum), zucchini.

- Grains: fonio, amaranth, Khorasan wheat (kamut), rye, wild rice, spelt, teff, quinoa.

- Nuts and Seeds: Brazil nuts, hemp seeds, crude sesame seeds, crude tahini spread, pecans.

- Oils: avocado oil, coconut oil (uncooked), grape seed oil, hempseed oil, olive oil (uncooked), sesame oil.

- Herbal teas: elderberry, chamomile, fennel, tila, burdock, ginger, raspberry.

- Spices: oregano, basil, cloves, inlet leaf, dill, sweet basil, achiote, cayenne, habanero, tarragon, onion powder, savvy, unadulterated ocean salt, thyme, powdered granulated kelp, unadulterated agave syrup, date sugar.

Notwithstanding tea, you are permitted to drink water.

Additionally, you may eat allowed grains as pasta, oat, bread or flour. Nonetheless, any food raised with yeast or preparing powder is prohibited.

In summary

This eating routine has an extremely exacting rundown of permitted nourishments. Nourishments that are excluded from this rundown ought to be evaded.

CHAPTER SEVEN

FOODS TO AVOID

Any nourishment that are excluded from the Dr. Sebi nourishment control are not allowed, for example,

- canned fruits or vegetables
- seedless fruits
- eggs
- dairy
- fish
- red meat
- poultry
- soy items
- processed food, including take-out or café food
- fortified nourishments

- wheat

- sugar (other than date sugar and agave syrup)

- alcohol

- yeast or nourishments ascended with yeast

- foods made with preparing powder

Moreover, numerous vegetables, fruits, grains, nuts, and seeds are restricted on the eating routine.

Just nourishments recorded in the guide might be eaten.

Outline

The eating routine restricts any food that is prepared, animal based, or made with leavening agents. Certain vegetables, fruits, grains, nuts, and seeds are not permitted.

CHAPTER EIGHT

DR SEBI SAMPLE MENU

Here is a three-day test menu on the Dr. Sebi diet.

Day 1

- Breakfast: 2 banana-spelt hotcakes with agave syrup

- Snack: 1 cup (240 ml) of green juice smoothie made with cucumbers, kale, apples, and ginger

- Lunch: kale serving of mixed greens with tomatoes, onions, avocado, dandelion greens, and chickpeas with olive oil and basil dressing

- Snack: home grown tea with fruits

- Dinner: vegetable and wild-rice pan sear

Day 2

- Breakfast: shake made with water, hemp seeds, bananas, and strawberries

- Snack: blueberry biscuits made with blueberries, unadulterated coconut milk, agave syrup, ocean salt, oil, and teff and spelt flour

- Lunch: hand crafted pizza utilizing a spelt-flour hull, Brazil-nut cheddar, and your selection of vegetables

- Snack: tahini spread on rye bread with cut red peppers as an afterthought

- Dinner: chickpea burger with tomato, onion, and kale on spelt-flour flatbread

Day 3

- Breakfast: cooked quinoa with agave syrup, peaches, and unadulterated coconut milk

- Snack: chamomile tea, cultivated grapes, and sesame seeds

- Lunch: spelt-pasta plate of mixed greens with hacked vegetables and an olive oil and key lime dressing

- Snack: a smoothie made with mango, banana, and unadulterated coconut milk

- Dinner: healthy vegetable soup utilizing mushrooms, red peppers, zucchini, onions, kale, flavors, water, and powdered ocean growth

In summary

This sample food plan centers on the endorsed fixings or ingredients that is added in the food guide. Dinners on this arrangement underline vegetables and fruits with modest quantities of the other nutrition types.

The Bottom Line

The Dr. Sebi diet stresses on eating entire, natural, plant-based food.

It might help weight reduction in the event that you don't typically eat in this manner.

Notwithstanding, it vigorously depends on taking the creator's costly supplements, is extremely prohibitive, does not have certain supplements, and mistakenly vows to change your body to an alkaline state.

In case you're hoping to follow a more plant-based eating design, numerous solid eating routine are more adaptable and feasible.

CHAPTER NINE

DR SEBI FOOD LIST

Dr. Sebi Vegetable List

Likewise with all his electric nourishments, Dr. Sebi believed that individuals ought to eat non-GMO nourishments. This incorporates foods grown from the ground that have been made seedless, or changed to contain a bigger number of nutrients and minerals than they do normally. The Dr. Sebi rundown of vegetables is somewhat enormous and various, with a lot of choices to make distinctive unique dinners. This rundown incorporates:

- Amaranth
- Arame

- Avocado
- Bell Pepper
- Chayote
- Cherry and Plum Tomato
- Cucumber
- Dandelion Greens
- Dulse
- Garbanzo Beans
- Hijiki
- Izote flower and leaf
- Kale
- Lettuce aside from ice shelf
- Mushrooms aside from Shitake
- Nopales
- Nori

- Okra
- Olives
- Onions
- Purslane Verdolaga
- Sea Vegetables
- Squash
- Tomatillo
- Turnip Greens
- Wakame
- Watercress
- Wild Arugula
- Zucchini

Dr. Sebi Fruit List

While the vegetable rundown is tolerably long, the fruits list is more limited, and numerous kinds of fruits aren't permitted to be burned-through while on the Dr. Sebi diet. Notwithstanding, the fruits list is still offers adherents of the eating routine an assorted arrangement of choices. For instance, all assortments of berries are permitted on the Dr. Sebi food list aside from cranberries, which are an artificial fruits. The rundown additionally incorporates:

- Apples
- Bananas
- Berries
- Cantaloupe
- Cherries
- Currants
- Dates
- Figs

- Grapes
- Limes
- Mango
- Melons
- Orange
- Papayas
- Peaches
- Pears
- Plums
- Prickly Pear
- Prunes
- Rasins
- Soft Jelly Coconuts
- Soursoups
- Tamarind

Dr Sebi Food List Spices and Seasonings

- Achiote
- Basil
- Bay Leaf

- Cayenne
- Cloves
- Dill
- Habanero
- Onion Powder
- Oregano
- Powdered Granulated Seaweed
- Pure Sea Salt
- Sage

- Savory
- Sweet Basil
- Tarragon
- Thyme

Basic or Alkaline Grains

- Amaranth
- Fonio
- Kamut
- Quinoa
- Rye
- Spelt
- Tef
- Wild Rice

Basic Sugars and Sweeteners

- Date Sugar from dried dates

- 100% Pure Agave Syrup from desert flora

Dr Sebi Herbal Teas

- Burdock
- Chamomile
- Elderberry
- Fennel
- Ginger
- Red Raspberry
- Tila

Nuts and Seeds

- Walnuts
- Brazil Nuts
- Hemp seeds
- Raw Sesame Seeds

Oils

- Olive Oil
- Coconut Oil
- Grapeseed Oil
- **Sesame Oil**
- Hempseed Oil
- Avocado Oil

IN CONCLUSION

A few weight watchers consider the Dr Sebi food rundown to be excessively restricting for their preferring. Nonetheless, dependable adherents of the eating regimen feel that there are sufficient nourishments on the rundown to take into account t assortment. A characteristic meal of the Dr. Sebi diet may look something like vegetables sauteed in avocado oil on a bed of wild rice, or a huge green plate of mixed greens with an olive oil dressing and a bit of agave syrup. Despite the fact that it might take some becoming accustomed to, the Dr. Sebi's food rundown can be anything but difficult to hold fast to and advantageous to one's wellbeing.

Made in the USA
Monee, IL
08 June 2022

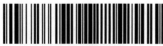